THIS JOURNAL BELONGS TO:

Ring The Bell
I Am Cancer Free

BELIEVE

COURAGE

STRONG

WARRIOR

SURVIVOR

FAITH

HEALED

_____

_____

_____

_____

_____

_____

_____

_____

_____

_____

_____

_____

_____

_____

_____

_____

_____

_____

_____

_____

_____

HOPE

FIGHTER

LOVE

JOY

DETERMINED

www.ingramcontent.com/pod-product-compliance
Lightning Source LLC
Chambersburg PA
CBHW020543220526
45463CB00006B/2177